Delicious Plant Based Cookbook

An Innovative Cooking Guide for New Meals

Jason Noel

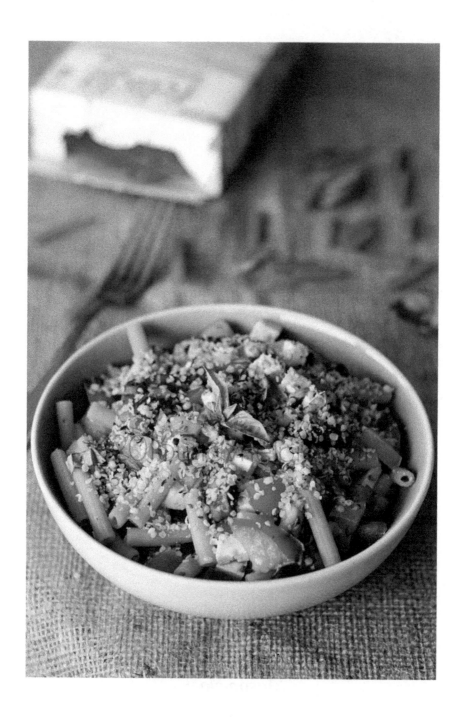

TABLE OF CONTENTS

Basil Spaghetti Pasta

Preparation Time: 05 minutes | Cooking Time: 05 minutes | Servings: 2

Ingredients:

- ½ teaspoon garlic powder
- 1 cup spaghetti
- 2 large eggs
- ¼ cup grated Parmesan cheese
- Freshly cracked pepper
- Salt and pepper to taste
- Handful fresh basil
- Enough water

Directions:

1. In a medium bowl, whisk together the eggs, 1/2 cup of the Parmesan cheese, and a generous dose of freshly cracked pepper.
2. Add spaghetti, water, basil, garlic powder, pepper, and salt to Pressure pot.
3. Place lid on Pressure pot and lock into place to seal.
4. Pressure Cook on High Pressure for 4 minutes.

5. Use Quick Pressure Release.

6. Pour the eggs and Parmesan mixture over the hot pasta.

Nutrition:

Calories216 | Total Fat 2. 3g | Saturated Fat 0. 7g | Cholesterol 49mg | Sodium 160mg | Total Carbohydrate 36g | Dietary Fiber 0. 1g | Total Sugars 0. 4g | Protein 12. 2g

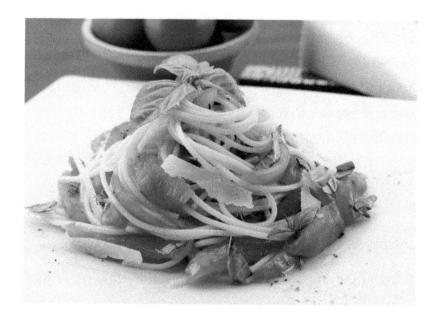

Parsley Hummus Pasta

Ingredients:

- ½ cup chickpeas
- 1/8 cup coconut oil
- ½ fresh lemon
- 1/8 cup tahini
- ½ teaspoon garlic powder
- 1/8 teaspoon cumin
- 1/4 teaspoon salt
- 1 green onion
- 1/8 bunch fresh parsley, or to taste
- 1 cup pasta
- Enough water

Directions:

1. Drain the chickpeas and add them to a food processor along with the coconut oil, juice from the lemon, tahini, garlic powder, cumin, and salt.
2. Pulse the ingredients, adding a small amount of water if needed to keep it moving, until the hummus is smooth.
3. Slice the green onion (both white and green ends) and pull the parsley leaves from the stems.

4. Add the green onion and parsley to the hummus in the food processor and process again until only small flecks of green remain.

5. Taste the hummus and adjust the salt, lemon, or garlic if needed.

6. Add pasta, water into Pressure pot.

7. Place the lid on the pot and lock it into place to seal.

8. Pressure Cook on High Pressure for 4 minutes.

9. Use Quick Pressure Release.

10. In Sauté mode add hummus to pasta.

11. When it mixes, turn off the switch of Pressure pot.

12. Serve and enjoy.

Nutrition:

• Calories 582 | Total Fat 26. 3g | Saturated Fat 13. 5g | Cholesterol 47mg | Sodium 338mg | Total Carbohydrate 71g | Dietary Fiber 10. 8g | Total Sugars 6. 1g | Protein 19. 9g

Creamy Spinach Artichoke Pasta

Preparation Time: 05 minutes | Cooking Time: 05 minutes | Servings: 2

Ingredients:

- 1 tablespoon butter
- ¼ teaspoon garlic powder
- 1 cup vegetable broth
- 1 cup of coconut milk
- ¼ teaspoon salt
- Freshly cracked pepper
- ½ cup pasta
- 1/4 cup fresh baby spinach
- ½ cup quartered artichoke hearts
- 1/8 cup grated Parmesan cheese

Directions:

1. In the Pressure pot, hit —Sauté‖, add butter when it melts, add garlic powder just until it's tender and fragrant.
2. Add the vegetable broth, coconut milk, salt, some freshly cracked pepper, and pasta.

3. Place the lid on the pot and lock it into place to seal.

4. Pressure Cook on High Pressure for 4 minutes.

5. Use Quick Pressure Release.

6. Add the spinach, a handful at a time, to the hot pasta and toss it in the pasta until it wilts into

7. Pressure pot in Sauté mode. Stir the chopped artichoke hearts into the pasta.

8. Sprinkle grated Parmesan over the pasta, then stir slightly to incorporate the Parmesan.

9. Top with an additional Parmesan then serve.

Nutrition:

Calories 457 | Total Fat 36. 2g | Saturated Fat 29. 6g | Cholesterol 40mg, Sodium 779mg | Total Carbohydrate 27. 6g | Dietary Fiber 4g | Total Sugars 4. 7g | Protein 10. 3g

Easy Spinach Ricotta Pasta

Preparation Time: 05 minutes | Cooking Time: 10 minutes | Servings: 2

Ingredients:

- ½ cup pasta
- 1 cup vegetable broth
- 1/2 lb. uncooked tagliatelle
- 1 tablespoon coconut oil
- ½ teaspoon garlic powder
- ¼ cup almond milk
- ½ cup whole milk ricotta
- 1/8 teaspoon salt
- Freshly cracked pepper
- ¼ cup chopped spinach

Directions:

1. Add the vegetable broth, tagliatelle, spinach, salt, some freshly cracked pepper, and the pasta.
2. Place lid on Pressure pot and lock into place to seal.
3. Pressure Cook on High Pressure for 4 minutes.
4. Use Quick Pressure Release.

5. Prepare the ricotta sauce.
6. Mince the garlic and add it to a large skillet with coconut oil.
7. Cook over Medium-Low heat for 1-2 minutes, or just until soft and fragrant (but not browned).
8. Add the almond milk and ricotta, then stir until relatively smooth (the ricotta may be slightly grainy).
9. Allow the sauce to heat through and come to a low simmer.
10. The sauce will thicken slightly as it simmers.
11. Once it's thick enough to coat the spoon (3-5 minutes), season with salt and pepper.
12. Add the cooked and drained pasta to the sauce and toss to coat.
13. If the sauce becomes too thick or dry, add a small amount of the reserved pasta cooking water.
14. Serve warm.

Nutrition:

Calories277 | Total Fat 18. 9g | Saturated Fat 15. 2g | Cholesterol 16mg |, Sodium 191mg, Total

Roasted Red Pepper Pasta

Preparation Time: 05 minutes | Cooking Time: 05 minutes | Servings: 2

Ingredients:

- 2 cups vegetable broth
- ½ cup spaghetti
- 1 small onion
- ½ teaspoon garlic minced
- ½ cup roasted red peppers
- ½ cup roasted diced tomatoes
- ¼ tablespoon dried mint
- 1/8 teaspoon crushed red pepper
- Freshly cracked black pepper
- ½ cup goat cheese

Directions:

1. In an Pressure pot, combine the vegetable broth, onion, garlic, red pepper slices, diced tomatoes, mint, crushed red pepper, and some freshly cracked black pepper.
2. Stir these ingredients to combine.
3. Add spaghetti to the Pressure pot.

4. Place lid on Pressure pot and lock into place to seal.

5. Pressure Cook on High Pressure for 4 minutes.

6. Use Quick Pressure Release.

7. Divide the goat cheese into tablespoon-sized pieces, then add them to the Pressure pot.

8. Stir the pasta until the cheese melts in and creates a smooth sauce.

9. Serve hot.

Nutrition:

Calories198 | Total Fat 4. 9g | Saturated Fat 2. 2g | Cholesterol 31mg | Sodium 909mg | Total Carbohydrate 26. 8g | Dietary Fiber 1. 9g | Total Sugars 5. 6g | Protein 11. 9g

Cheese Beetroot Greens Macaroni

Preparation Time: 05 minutes | Cooking Time: 05 minutes | Servings: 2

Ingredients:

- 1 tablespoon butter
- 1 clove garlic minced
- 1 cup button mushrooms
- ½ bunch beetroot greens
- ½ cup vegetable broth
- ½ cup macaroni
- ¼ teaspoon salt
- ½ cup grated Parmesan cheese
- Freshly cracked pepper

Directions:

1. In the Pressure pot, hit ─Sauté‖, add butter, garlic and slice the mushrooms.
2. Add the beetroot greens to the pot along with 1/2 cup vegetable broth.

3. Stir the beetroot greens as it cooks until it is fully wilted.

4. Add vegetable broth, macaroni, salt, and pepper.

5. Place lid on Pressure pot and lock into place to seal.

6. Pressure Cook on High Pressure for 4 minutes.

7. Use Quick Pressure Release.

8. Add grated Parmesan cheese.

Nutrition:

Calories 147 | Total Fat 8g | Saturated Fat 4. 8g | Cholesterol 23mg | Sodium 590mg | Total Carbohydrate 12. 7g | Dietary Fiber 1g | Total Sugars 1. 5g | Protein 6. 5g

Pastalaya

Preparation Time: 05 minutes | Cooking Time: 05 minutes | Servings: 2

Ingredients:

- ½ tablespoon avocado oil
- ½ teaspoon garlic powder
- 1 diced tomato
- ¼ teaspoon dried basil
- ¼ teaspoon smoked paprika
- ¼ teaspoon dried rosemary
- Freshly cracked pepper
- 1 cup vegetable broth
- ½ cup of water
- 1 cup orzo pasta
- 1 tablespoon coconut cream
- ½ bunch fresh coriander

Directions:

1. In the Pressure pot, place the garlic powder and avocado oil, sauté for 15 seconds, or until the garlic is fragrant.

2. Add diced tomatoes, basil, smoked paprika, rosemary, freshly cracked pepper, and orzo pasta to the Pressure pot.
3. Finally, add the vegetable broth and ½ cup of water, and stir until everything is evenly combined.
4. Place the lid on the Pressure pot, and bring the toggle switch into the −Sealing‖ position.
5. Press Manual or Pressure Cook and adjust the time for 5 minutes.
6. When the five minutes are up, do a Natural-release for 5 minutes and then move the toggle switch to −Venting‖ to release the rest of the pressure in the pot.
7. Remove the lid.
8. If the mixturelooks watery, press −Sauté‖ and bring the mixture up to a boil and let it boil for a few minutes. It will thicken as it boils.
9. Add the coconut cream and leek to the Pressure pot, stir and let warm through for a few minutes.
10. Serve and garnish with coriander toast. Enjoy!

Nutrition:

Calories 351 | Total Fat 6. 8g | Saturated Fat 3. 5g | Cholesterol 56mg | Sodium 869mg

Pasta with Peppers

Preparation Time: 5 minutes | Cooking Time: 15 minutes | Servings: 2

Ingredients:

- 1 1/2 cups spaghetti sauce
- 1 cup vegetable broth
- ½ tablespoon dried Italian seasoning blend
- 1 cup bell pepper strips
- 1 cup dried pasta
- 1 cup shredded Romano cheese

Directions:

1. Press the button Sauté.
2. Set it for High, and set the time for 10 minutes.
3. Mix the sauce, broth, and seasoning blend in a Pressure pot. Cook, turn off the Sauté
4. function; stir in the bell pepper strips and pasta.
5. Lock the lid onto the pot.
6. Press Pressure Cook on Max Pressure for 5 minutes with the Keep Warm setting off.

7. Use the Quick Release method to bring the pot pressure back to normal.
8. Unlatch the lid and open the cooker.
9. Stir in the shredded Romano cheese.
10. Set the lid askew over the pot and set aside for 5 minutes to melt the cheese and let the pasta continue to absorb excess liquid.
11. Serve by the big spoon.

Nutrition:

Calories 291 | Total Fat 6. 2g | Saturated Fat 2. 9g | Cholesterol 61mg | Sodium 994mg | Total Carbohydrate 43. 7g | Dietary Fiber 1g | Total Sugars 3. 5g | Protein 15. 1g

Fresh Tomato Mint Pasta

Preparation Time: 05 minutes | Cooking Time: 10 minutes | Servings: 2

Ingredients:

- 1 cup pasta
- 1 tablespoon coconut oil
- ½ teaspoon garlic powder
- 1 tomato
- ½ tablespoon butter
- ¼ cup fresh mint
- ¼ cup of coconut milk
- Salt & pepper to taste
- Enough water

Directions:

1. Add the coconut oil to the Pressure pot hit —Sauté‖, add in the garlic, and stir.
2. Add the tomatoes and a pinch of salt.
3. Then add mint and pepper.
4. Next, add coconut milk, butter, and water.
5. Stir well, lastly, add in the pasta.

6. Secure the lid and hit ─Keep Warm/Cancel‖ and then hit ─Manual‖ or ─Pressure Cook‖ High Pressure for 6 minutes.
7. Quick-release when done.
8. Enjoy.

Nutrition:

Calories 350 | Total Fat 18. 5g | Saturated Fat 14. 3g | Cholesterol 54mg | Sodium 47mg | Total Carbohydrate 39. 4g | Dietary Fiber 1. 9g | Total Sugars 2g | Protein 8. 7g

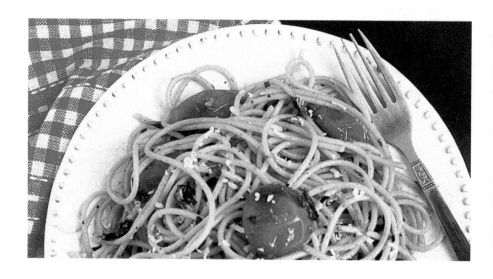

Corn and Chiles Fusilli

Preparation Time: 05 minutes | Cooking Time: 05 minutes | Servings: 2

Ingredients:

- ½ tablespoon butter
- 1 tablespoon garlic minced
- Salt and pepper to taste
- 2 oz. can green chills
- ½ cup frozen corn kernels
- ¼ teaspoon cumin
- 1/8 teaspoon paprika
- 1 cup fusilli
- 1 cup vegetable broth
- ¼ cup coconut cream
- 2 leeks, sliced
- 1/8 bunch parsley
- 1 oz. shredded mozzarella cheese

Directions:

1. In the Pressure pot, add butter when butter melt, place the minced garlic, salt, and pepper, then press Sauté on the Pressure pot.

2. Add the can of green chills (with juices), frozen corn kernels, cumin, and paprika.

3. Add the uncooked fusilli and vegetable broth to the Pressure pot.

4. Place the lid on the Pressure pot, and bring the toggle switch into the −Sealing‖ position.

5. Press Manual or Pressure Cook and adjust the time for 5 minutes.

6. When the five minutes are up, do a Natural-release for 5 minutes and then move the toggle switch to −Venting‖ to release the rest of the pressure in the pot.

7. Remove the lid.

8. If the mixture looks watery, press −Sauté‖, and bring the mixture up to a boil and let it boil for a few minutes.

9. Then add the coconut cream and stir until it has fully coated the pasta.

10. Stir in most of the sliced leek and parsley, reserving a little to sprinkle over top, mozzarella on top of the pasta.

Nutrition:

Calories 399 | Total Fat 14. 4g | Saturated Fat 10g | Cholesterol 15mg | Sodium 531mg | Total Carbohydrate 56. 2g | Dietary Fiber 4. 9g |Total Sugars 7. 2g | Protein 15. 4g

Creamy Penne with Vegetables

• Preparation Time: 05 minutes | Cooking Time: 10 minutes | Servings: 2

Ingredients:

- ½ tablespoon butter
- 1 cup penne
- 1 small onion
- ½ teaspoon garlic powder
- 1 carrot
- ½ red bell pepper
- ½ pumpkin
- 2 cups vegetable broth
- 2 oz. coconut cream
- 1/8 cup grated Parmesan cheese
- 1/8 teaspoon salt and pepper to taste
- Dash hot sauce, optional
- ¼ cup cauliflower florets

Directions:

1. Set Pressure pot to Sauté.
2. Add the butter and allow it to melt.

3. Add the onion and garlic powder and cook for 2 minutes.
4. Stir regularly.
5. Add the carrot, red pepper and pumpkin, and cauliflower to the pot.
6. Add penne, vegetable broth, coconut cream, salt, and pepper then add hot sauce.
7. Lock the lid and make sure the vent is closed.
8. Set Pressure pot to Manual or Pressure Cook on High Pressure for 10 minutes.
9. When cooking time ends, release pressure and wait for steam to completely stop before opening the lid.
10. Stir in cheese, sprinkle a bit on top of the pasta when you serve it.

Nutrition:

Calories 381 | Total Fat 13. 2g | Saturated Fat 8. 7g | Cholesterol 56mg | Sodium 1006mg | Total Carbohydrate 52. 3g | Dietary Fiber 4. 7g | Total Sugars 8. 6g | Protein 15. 3g

Pasta with Eggplant Sauce

Preparation Time: 05 minutes | Cooking Time: 10 minutes | Servings: 2

Ingredients:

- 1 tablespoon coconut oil
- 2 cloves garlic
- 1 small onion
- 1 medium eggplant
- 1 cup diced tomatoes
- 1 tablespoon tomato sauce
- ¼ teaspoon dried thyme
- ½ teaspoon honey
- Pinch paprika
- Freshly cracked pepper
- ¼ salt and pepper, or to taste
- 6 oz. spaghetti
- 2 cups vegetable broth
- Handful fresh coriander, chopped

Directions:

1. Set Pressure pot to Sauté.

2. Add the coconut oil and allow it to melt.

3. Add the onion and garlic and cook for 2 minutes or until the onion is soft and transparent.

4. Add eggplant, diced tomatoes, tomato sauce, thyme, honey, paprika, and freshly cracked pepper.

5. Stir them well to combine.

6. Add spaghetti, and vegetable broth, salt, and pepper.

7. Lock the lid and make sure the vent is closed.

8. Set Pressure pot to Manual or Pressure Cook on High Pressure for 10 minutes.

9. When cooking time ends, release pressure and wait for steam to completely stop before opening the lid.

10. Top each serving with grated goat and a sprinkle of fresh coriander.

Nutrition:

Calories 306 | Total Fat 18g | Saturated Fat 12. 9g | Cholesterol 30mg | Sodium 188mg | Total Carbohydrate 27g | Dietary Fiber 12. 6g 45% | Total Sugars 13. 9g | Protein 14. 2g

Creamy Pesto Pasta With Tofu & Broccoli

Preparation Time: 05 minutes | Cooking Time: 10 minutes | Servings: 2

Ingredients:

- 4 oz. Farfalle pasta
- 4 oz. frozen broccoli florets
- ½ tablespoon coconut oil
- ½ cup tofu
- ¼ cup basil pesto
- ¼ cup vegetable broth
- 2 oz. heavy cream

Directions:

1. In the Pressure pot, add Farfalline pasta, broccoli, coconut oil, tofu, basil pesto, vegetable broth.
2. Cover the Pressure pot and lock it in.
3. Set the Manual or Pressure Cook timer for 10 minutes.
4. Make sure the timer is set to −Sealing‖.

5. Once the timer reaches zero, quickly release the pressure. Add heavy cream.

6. Enjoy.

Nutrition:

Calories 383 | Total Fat 17. 8g | Saturated Fat 10. 1g | Cholesterol 39mg | Sodium 129mg | Total Carbohydrate 44g | Dietary Fiber 2. 4g | Total Sugars 3. 2g | Protein 13. 6g

Chili Cheese Cottage Cheese Mac

Preparation Time: 05 minutes | Cooking Time: 12 minutes | Servings: 2

Ingredients:

- ½ tablespoon butter
- 1 cup cottage cheese
- ½ teaspoon garlic powder
- 1 small onion
- 1 tablespoon coconut flour
- ½ tablespoon chili powder
- ¼ teaspoon smoked paprika
- ¼ teaspoon dried basil
- 1 cup tomato paste
- 2 cups vegetable broth
- 1 cup dry macaroni
- ½ cup shredded sharp cheddar

Directions:

1. Set the Pressure pot to Sauté.
2. Add butter and wait one minute to heat up.
3. Add the cottage cheese, sauté for one minute.

4. Stir often.

5. Add coconut flour, onion, and garlic powder.

6. Add the chili powder, smoked paprika, basil, tomato paste, and 2 cups of vegetable broth.

7. Add the dry macaroni and cottage cheese.

8. Stir well.

9. Cover the Pressure pot and lock it in.

10. Set the Manual or Pressure Cook timer for 10 minutes.

11. Make sure the timer is set to—Sealing‖.

12. Once the timer reaches zero, quickly release the pressure.

13. Add shredded sharp cheddar cheese and enjoy.

Nutrition:

Calories 509 | Total Fat 11. 3g | Saturated Fat 6. 4g | Cholesterol 23mg | Sodium 1454mg | Total Carbohydrate 70. 3g | Dietary Fiber 10. 8g | Total Sugars 20. 5g | Protein 34. 8g

Spicy Cauliflower Pasta

Preparation Time: 05 minutes | Cooking Time: 10 minutes | Servings: 2

Ingredients:

- 1 tablespoon coconut oil
- 1 teaspoon garlic powder
- ¼ teaspoon paprika
- ½ cup cauliflower florets
- ½ cup broccoli florets
- 1 cup bow tie pasta
- Salt & pepper to taste
- 1 cup vegetable broth

Directions:

1. In the Pressure pot, set the Sauté button and add coconut oil when oil is hot, place garlic powder, paprika, cauliflower florets, broccoli florets, salt, and pepper.
2. Sauté the mixture untilit's cooked thoroughly.
3. Add the vegetable broth, and dry bow tie pasta.
4. Mix very well and place the lid on the Pressure pot, and bring the toggle switch into the −Sealing‖ position.

5. Press Manual or Pressure Cook and adjust the time for 5 minutes.

6. When the five minutes are up, do a Natural-release for 5 minutes and then move the toggle switch to ―Venting‖ to release the rest of the pressure in the pot.

7. Remove the lid. If the mixture looks watery, press ―Sauté‖, and bring the mixture up to a boil and let it boil for a few minutes. It will thicken as it boils.

8. Serve and enjoy!

Nutrition:

Calories298 | Total Fat 10. 4g | Saturated Fat 7. 2g | Cholesterol 50mg | Sodium 426mg | Total Carbohydrate 39. 6g | Dietary Fiber 1. 5g | Total Sugars 1. 8g |Protein 12. 2g

Tasty Mac and Cheese

Preparation Time: 05 minutes | Cooking Time: 10 minutes |
Servings: 2

Ingredients:

- ½ cup of soy milk
- 1 cup dry macaroni
- Enough water
- ½ cup shredded mozzarella cheese
- ¼ teaspoon salt
- ¼ teaspoon Dijon mustard
- 1/8 teaspoon red chili powder

Directions:

1. Add macaroni, soy milk, water, and salt, chili powder, Dijon mustard to the Pressure pot.
2. Place lid on Pressure pot and lock into place to seal.
3. Pressure Cook on High Pressure for 4 minutes.
4. Use Quick Pressure Release.
5. Stir cheese into macaroni and then stir in the cheeses until melted and combined.

Nutrition:

Calories 210 | Total Fat 3g, Saturated Fat 1g | Cholesterol 4mg | Sodium 374mg | Total Carbohydrate 35. 7g | Dietary Fiber 1. 8g | Total Sugars 3. 6g | Protein 9. 6g

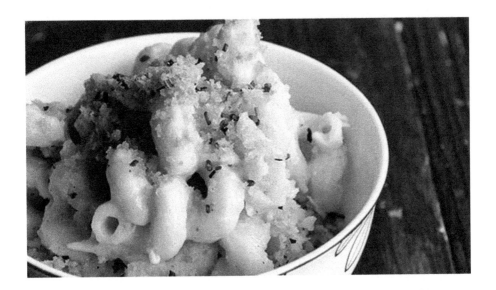

Jackfruit and Red Pepper Pasta

• Preparation Time: 05 minutes | Cooking Time: 17 minutes | Servings: 2

Ingredients:

- ½ cup gnocchi
- 1/8 cup avocado oil
- ½ tablespoon garlic powder
- 1/2 teaspoon crushed red pepper
- ½ bunch fresh mint
- ½ cup jackfruit
- Salt to taste
- Enough water

Directions:

1. Set Pressure pot to Sauté.
2. Add the avocado oil and allow it to sizzle.
3. Add the garlic powder and cook for 2 minutes.
4. Stir regularly.
5. Add jackfruit and cook until about 4 - 5 minutes.
6. Add gnocchi, water, fresh mint, salt, and red pepper into Pressure pot.

7. Lock the lid and make sure the vent is closed.

8. Set Pressure pot to Manual or Pressure Cook on High PRESSURE for 10 minutes.

9. When cooking time ends, release pressure and wait for steam to completely stop before opening the lid.

10. Enjoy.

Nutrition:

Calories 110 | Total Fat 2. 3g | Saturated Fat 0. 4g | Cholesterol 0mg | Sodium 168mg | Total Carbohydrate 21. 5g | Dietary Fiber 2. 5g | Total Sugars 0. 6g | Protein 2. 3g

Creamy Mushroom Pasta with Broccoli

Preparation Time: 05 minutes | Cooking Time: 12 minutes | Servings: 2

Ingredients:

- 1 tablespoon coconut oil
- 1 small onion
- ½ teaspoon garlic powder
- 1 cup mushrooms
- 1 tablespoon coconut flour
- 1 cup of water
- ¼ cup red wine
- 1/8 cup coconut cream
- ¼ teaspoon dried basil
- Salt and pepper to taste
- 1/8 bunch fresh cilantro
- ½ cup mozzarella cheese
- 4 oz. pasta
- ½ cup broccoli

Directions:

1. Set Pressure pot to Sauté.
2. Add the coconut oil and allow it to sizzle.
3. Add coconut flour and mushrooms, sauté for 2 minutes.
4. Stir regularly.
5. It will coat the mushrooms and will begin to turn golden in color.
6. Just make sure to keep stirring so that the flour does not burn.
7. Combine water along with the red wine, basil, salt, and pepper.
8. Whisk until no flour lumps remain.
9. Add pasta, broccoli, cilantro, onion, and garlic powder.
10. Lock the lid and make sure the vent is closed.
11. Set Pressure pot to Manual or Pressure Cook on High Pressure for 10 minutes.
12. cooking time ends, release pressure and wait for steam to completely stop before opening the lid.
13. Stir in cheese and coconut cream.
14. Serve hot and enjoy.

Nutrition:

• Calories 363 | Total Fat 14. 2g | Saturated Fat 11g | Cholesterol 45mg | Sodium 91mg | Total Carbohydrate 43. 4g | Dietary Fiber 4. 6g | Total Sugars 3. 9g | Protein 12. 1g

Peanut Noodles Stir Fry

Preparation Time: 05 minutes | Cooking Time: 17 minutes | Servings: 2

Ingredients:

- ½ teaspoon ginger powder
- ¼ cup natural peanut butter
- ¼ cup hoisin sauce
- 1 cup hot water
- ¼ teaspoon sriracha hot sauce
- 1 tablespoon vegetable oil
- ½ teaspoon garlic powder
- 1 cup frozen stir fry vegetables
- 2 oz. soba noodles
- 2 sliced leek, optional

Directions:

1. Prepare the sauce first.
2. Add ginger powder into a bowl.
3. Add the peanut butter, hoisin sauce, sriracha hot sauce, and ¼ cup of hot water.
4. Stir or whisk until smooth.

44

5. Set the sauce aside until it is needed.

6. Set the Pressure pot to Sauté.

7. Add the vegetable oil and allow it to sizzle.

8. Add garlic powder and ginger powder and cook for 2 minutes.

9. Add the bag of frozen vegetables and cook for 5 minutes.

10. Add the remaining water and soba noodles.

11. Lock the lid and make sure the vent is closed.

12. Set Pressure pot to Manual or Pressure Cook on High Pressure for 10 minutes.

13. When cooking time ends, release pressure and wait for steam to completely stop before opening the lid.

14. Stir until everything is combined and coated with sauce.

15. Garnish with sliced leek if desired.

Nutrition:

Calories 501 | Total Fat 24. 4g | Saturated Fat 4. 6g | Cholesterol 1mg | Sodium 788mg | Total Carbohydrate 58. 1g | Dietary Fiber 6g | Total Sugars 15. 8g | Protein 17. 3g

Cauliflower Shells Cheese

Preparation Time: 05 minutes | Cooking Time: 15 minutes | Servings: 2

Ingredients:

- 4 oz. macaroni
- 1 cup vegetable broth
- ½ cup cauliflower florets
- 1/2 small onion
- 1 1/2 tablespoons butter
- 1 1/2 tablespoons coconut flour
- 1 1/2 cups coconut milk
- 1 cup sharp cheddar, shredded
- Salt and pepper to taste

Directions:

1. Set the Pressure pot to Sauté, add the coconut flour, butter, and onion.
2. The flour and butter will form a paste, whisk for 1-2 minutes more taking care not to let it scorch.

3. This slightly cooks the flour preventing the cheese sauce from having an overly strong flour flavor or paste-like flavor.
4. Whisk the milk into the roux until no lumps remain.
5. Add some freshly cracked pepper to the sauce.
6. Bring the mixture up to a simmer, stirring often.
7. Set aside.
8. Add macaroni and vegetable broth into Pressure pot.
9. Lock the lid and make sure the vent is closed.
10. Add cauliflower and set Pressure pot to Manual or Pressure Cook on High Pressure for 10 minutes.
11. When cooking time ends, release pressure and wait for steam to completely stop before opening the lid.
12. Add cheddar and stir sauce mix well with macaroni.

Nutrition:

Calories 643 | Total Fat 53. 6g | Saturated Fat 42. 1g | Cholesterol 75mg | Sodium 443mg | Total Carbohydrate 26. 2g | Dietary Fiber 6. 6g | Total Sugars 6. 2g | Protein 18. 4g

Lemon Mozzarella Pasta

Preparation Time: 05 minutes | Cooking Time: 10 minutes | Servings: 2

Ingredients:

- 4 oz. macaroni
- ¼ cup peas
- ½ cup mozzarella cheese
- ½ tablespoon olive oil
- 1 lemon
- Salt and pepper

Directions:

1. Set Pressure pot to Sauté.
2. Add the olive oil and allow it to sizzle.
3. Add macaroni, peas, lemon, salt, and pepper.
4. Lock the lid and make sure the vent is closed.
5. Set Pressure pot to Manual or Pressure Cook on High Pressure for 10 minutes.
6. When cooking time ends, release pressure and wait for steam to completely stop before opening the lid.

7. Add mozzarella cheese and Stir until everything is combined and coated with sauce.

8. Enjoy.

Nutrition:

Calories 273 | Total Fat 5. 9g | Saturated Fat 1. 3g | Cholesterol 4mg | Sodium 44mg | Total Carbohydrate 46. 6g | Dietary Fiber 3. 7g | Total Sugars 2. 8g | Protein 10. 3g

Kale Lasagna Roll-Ups

Preparation Time: 10 minutes | Cooking Time: 15 minutes | Servings: 2

Ingredients:

- ½ cup Lasagna noodles
- ½ cup goat cheese
- ½ cup mozzarella, shredded
- 1 large egg
- ¼ cup kale
- ½ cup marinara sauce
- Salt and pepper to taste
- Enough water

Directions:

1. Set Pressure pot to Sauté.
2. Add the kale with goat cheese, mozzarella, egg, pepper, and salt.
3. Stir regularly.
4. Add marinara sauce, water, noodles.
5. Mix well.
6. Stir to make sure noodles are covered with the liquid.

7. Lock the lid and make sure the vent is closed.

8. Set Pressure pot to Manual or Pressure Cook on High Pressure for 15 minutes.

9. When cooking time ends, release pressure and wait for steam to completely stop before opening the lid.

10. If you would like to sprinkle a bit on top of the Lasagna when you serve it.

Nutrition:

Calories 343 | Total Fat 23. 6g | Saturated Fat 22. 1g | Cholesterol 17. 5mg | Sodium 243mg | Total Carbohydrate 16. 2g | Dietary Fiber 3. 6g | Total Sugars 2. 2g | Protein 16. 4g

Zucchini Noodles

Preparation Time: 10 minutes | Cooking Time: 15 minutes | Servings: 2

Ingredients:

- 2 zucchini, peeled
- Marinara sauce of your choice
- Any other seasonings you wish to use

Directions:

• Peel & spiralizer your zucchini into noodles.

1. Add some of your favorite sauce to Pressure pot, hit —Sauté‖ and —Adjust‖ so it's on the—More‖ or —High‖ setting.
2. Once the sauce is bubbling, add the noodles to the pot, toss them in the sauce, and allow them to heat up and soften for a few minutes for about 2-5 minutes.
3. Serve in bowls and top with some grated parmesan, if desired.
4. Enjoy!

Nutrition:

Calories 86 | Total Fat 2g | Saturated Fat 0. 5g | Cholesterol 1mg | Sodium 276mg | Total Carbohydrate 15. 2g | Dietary Fiber 3. 8g | Total Sugars 8. 9g | Protein 3. 5g

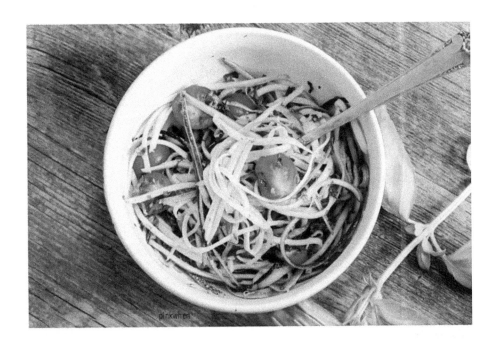

Lemon Parsley Pasta

Preparation Time: 10 minutes | Cooking Time: 15 minutes | Servings: 2

Ingredients:

- 1 cup ziti pasta
- ½ cup fresh parsley, finely chopped
- 1 lemon zest
- 1 teaspoon garlic powder
- 1 1/2 tablespoon coconut oil
- ½ tablespoon butter
- 2 tablespoon parmesan cheese
- Salt and fresh black pepper
- Enough water

Directions:

1. Add butter to the Pressure pot, hit —Sauté‖ and once the butter is melted and sizzled, Add parsley, lemon zest, garlic powder, coconut oil, salt, and black pepper.
2. Lock the lid and make sure the vent is closed.
3. Add water and ziti pasta. Set Pressure pot to Manual or Pressure Cook on High PRESSURE for 10 minutes.

4. When cooking time ends, release pressure and wait for steam to completely stop before opening the lid.
5. Stir in cheese.
6. Serve and enjoy.

Nutrition:

Calories 377 | Total Fat 17. 4g | Saturated Fat 11. 9g | Cholesterol 74mg | Sodium 306mg | Total Carbohydrate 40. 7g | Dietary Fiber 1. 5g | Total Sugars 1. 2g | Protein 17. 3g

Creamy Tofu Marsala Pasta

Preparation Time: 10 minutes | Cooking Time: 15 minutes | Servings: 2

Ingredients:

- ¼ cup butter
- 1 tablespoon coconut oil
- 1 small onion, diced
- 2 cup mushrooms, sliced
- ½ cup tofu, diced into chunks
- ½ teaspoon garlic powder
- 1 1/2 cups of vegetable broth
- 1 cup of white wine
- ½ cup sun-dried tomatoes
- 1 cup fusilli
- 1/4 cup coconut cream
- ½ cup grated goat cheese

Directions:

1. Add the butter to the Pressure pot.
2. Hit —Sauté‖.
3. Add the onion and mushrooms and cook for 3-5 minutes, until the mushrooms have softened and browned a bit.

4. Then, add the tofu and the coconut oil from the sun-dried tomatoes and cook for another 2-3 minutes until the tofu is slightly white.
5. Toss in the garlic powder and cook for 1 more minute and then add in the white wine and let it simmer for 1 minute more.
6. Add in the vegetable broth and stir together well.
7. Pour in the fusilli so it's laying on top of the broth, gently smoothing and pushing it down with a spatula so it's submerged, but do not stir it with the rest of the broth.
8. Secure the lid and hit —Manual‖ or —Pressure Cook‖ High Pressure for 6 minutes.
9. Quick- release when done and give it all a good stir.
10. Stir in the coconut cream and goat cheese.
11. Let it sit for about 5 minutes, stirring occasionally and it will thicken up into an incredible sauce, coating all the pasta perfectly.
12. Transfer to a serving bowl, plate it up, and sprinkle any extra goat cheese if desired.
13. Enjoy!

Nutrition:

Calories 510 | Total Fat 20. 6g | Saturated Fat 14. 8g | Cholesterol 7mg | Sodium 432mg | Total Carbohydrate 45. 9g | Dietary Fiber 4. 8g | Total Sugars 7. 8g | Protein 19. 1g

Classic Goulash

Preparation Time: 10 minutes | Cooking Time: 15 minutes | Servings: 2

Ingredients:

- 1 cup crumbled tofu
- 2 onions, chopped
- 1 teaspoon garlic powder
- 2 cups of water
- 1 cup tomato paste
- 1cup diced tomatoes
- 1 1/2 tablespoons soy sauce
- ½ tablespoon dried basil
- 1 bay leaf
- ¼ tablespoon seasoned salt, or to taste
- 1 cup uncooked elbow macaroni

Directions:

1. Set Pressure pot to Sauté. Add crumbled tofu.
2. Add the onions and garlic powder and cook for 2 minutes.
3. Stir regularly.

4. Stir water, tomato paste, diced tomatoes, soy sauce, dried basil, bay leaf, and seasoned salt

5. into the tofu mixture.

6. Stir macaroni into the mixture, Secure the lid, and hit —Manual‖ or —Pressure Cook‖ High

7. Pressure for 6 minutes.

8. Quick-release when done.

9. Enjoy.

Nutrition:

Calories 425 | Total Fat 7. 5g | Saturated Fat 1. 2g | Cholesterol 0mg | Sodium 647mg | Total Carbohydrate 73. 5g | Dietary Fiber 10. 7g | Total Sugars 24. 3g | Protein 23. 8g

Penne with Spicy Vodka Tomato Cream Sauce

Preparation Time: 10 minutes | Cooking Time: 15 minutes | Servings: 2

Ingredients:

- ½ cup uncooked penne pasta
- 1/8 cup coconut oil
- Enough water
- 1 teaspoon garlic powder
- ¼ teaspoon paprika
- ½ cup crushed tomatoes
- ½ teaspoon salt
- 1 tablespoon vodka
- ½ cup coconut cream
- 1/8 cup chopped fresh cilantro

Directions:

1. Add penne pasta, coconut oil, water, paprika, crushed tomatoes, vodka, garlic powder, and salt to Pressure pot.
2. Place the lid on the pot and lock it into place to seal.

3. Pressure Cook on High Pressure for 4 minutes.

4. Use Quick Pressure Release.

5. Stir coconut cream into penne pasta and then stir in the fresh cilantro and combine.

Nutrition:

Calories 394 |, Total Fat 28. 7g | Saturated Fat 24. 6g | Cholesterol 23mg | Sodium 720mg | Total Carbohydrate 27g | Dietary Fiber 3. 6g | Total Sugars 5. 9g | Protein 6. 8g

Creamy Pesto Tofu

Preparation Time: 10 minutes | Cooking Time: 15 minutes | Servings: 2

Ingredients:

- ½ cup vermicelli pasta
- ¼ cup butter
- 1/2 teaspoon ground black pepper
- ¼ cup grated mozzarella cheese
- ¼ cup basil pesto
- ½ cup tofu, peeled
- Enough water

Directions:

1. Set the Pressure pot to Sauté.
2. Add butter and wait one minute to heat up.
3. Add the tofu, basil pesto sauté for one minute.
4. Stir often.
5. Add water, vermicelli pasta, and pepper.
6. Place the lid on the pot and lock it into place to seal.
7. Pressure Cook on High Pressure for 4 minutes.
8. Use Quick Pressure Release.

9. Stir mozzarella cheese.

10. Serve and enjoy.

Nutrition:

Calories 711 | Total Fat 62. 3g | Saturated Fat 52. 7g | Cholesterol 15mg | Sodium 77mg | Total Carbohydrate 32. 5g | Dietary Fiber 6. 8g | Total Sugars 8. 8g | Protein 15. 6g

Garlic Lasagna

Preparation Time: 10 minutes | Cooking Time: 20min | Servings: 2

Ingredients:

- ½ tablespoon butter
- ½ tablespoon coconut oil
- 1 small onion chopped
- 1 tablespoon garlic powder
- ½ cup ground cauliflower
- ½ cup pasta sauce
- 2 cups vegetable broth
- 1/8 cup white wine
- 1 cup of water
- 1teaspoon Italian seasoning
- 1 cup uncooked Lasagna noodles
- ½ cup shredded goat cheese divided
- 1/4 cup Parmesan cheese

Directions:

1. Set Pressure pot to Sauté.
2. Add the coconut oil and butter and allow it to sizzle.

3. Add the onions and garlic powder and cook for 2 minutes.

4. Stir regularly.

5. Add ground cauliflower and cook until about 4 - 5 minutes into Pressure pot.

6. Add pasta sauce, vegetable broth, white wine, water, and Italian seasonings.

7. Mix well.

8. Add Lasagna noodles.

9. Stir to make sure noodles are covered with the liquid.

10. Lock the lid and make sure the vent is closed.

11. Set Pressure pot to Manual or Pressure Cook on high pressure for 10 minutes.

12. When cooking time ends, release pressure and wait for steam to completely stop before opening the lid.

13. Stir in goat cheese and Parmesan cheese, but reserve about 1/8 cup Parmesan cheese if you would like to sprinkle a bit on top of the Lasagna when you serve it.

Nutrition:

Calories 325 | Total Fat 13. 4g | Saturated Fat 7. 5g | Cholesterol 31mg | Sodium 1117mg | Total Carbohydrate 34. 5g | Dietary Fiber 3. 4g | Total Sugars 9. 7g | Protein 14g

Tomato Sauce with Pumpkin

Preparation Time: 10 minutes | Cooking Time: 15 minutes | Servings: 2

Ingredients:

- ½ cup avocado oil
- 1 small onion diced
- 1 teaspoon garlic minced
- 1 cup pumpkin
- 1/8 cup fresh coriander washed and chopped
- 1 cup crushed tomatoes
- 1 tablespoon tomato paste
- ½ tablespoon dried basil
- 1/2 teaspoon salt and pepper

Directions:

1. Set the Pressure pot to Sauté.
2. Add avocado oil and wait one minute to heat up.
3. Add the onion and garlic, sauté for one minute.
4. Stir often.
5. Add the pumpkin, coriander, and sauté for one minute.
6. Stir often.

7. Add the crushed tomatoes, tomato paste, dried basil, salt, and pepper.

8. Stir well.

9. Cover the Pressure pot and lock it in.

10. Set the Manual or Pressure Cook timer for 10 minutes.

11. Make sure the timer is set to—Sealing‖.

12. Once the timer reaches zero, quickly release the pressure.

13. Enjoy!

Nutrition:

Calories191 | Total Fat 7. 6g | Saturated Fat 1. 7g | Cholesterol 0mg | Sodium 840mg | Total Carbohydrate 28. 9g | Dietary Fiber 11. 4g | Total Sugars | Protein 6g

Eggplant Fettuccine Pasta

Preparation Time: 05 minutes | Cooking Time: 25 minutes | Servings: 2

Ingredients:

- 1 tablespoon coconut oil
- 1 onion finely diced
- 1 medium zucchini chopped
- 2 cloves garlic minced
- 1 tablespoon tomato paste
- 1/2 cup vegetable broth
- 1 teaspoon dried thyme
- 1 teaspoon dried oregano
- 1 teaspoon kosher salt
- ¼ teaspoon pepper
- ½ cup diced tomatoes
- 1 cup eggplant, diced
- 1 tablespoon corn-starch
- 1 cup juice
- Shredded goat cheese for garnish

Directions:

1. Add coconut oil to the Pressure pot.
2. Using the display panel select the Sauté function.

3. When oil gets hot, add onion to the Pressure pot and sauté for 3 minutes.
4. Add zucchini and cook for 3 minutes more.
5. Add garlic and tomato paste and cook for 1-2 minutes more.
6. Add vegetable broth and seasonings to the Pressure pot and deglaze by using a wooden spoon to scrape the brown bits from the bottom of the pot.
7. Add tomatoes to the Pressure pot and stir.
8. Add eggplant to the Pressure pot, turning once to coat.
9. Turn the Pressure pot off by selecting Cancel, then secure the lid, making sure the vent is closed.
10. Using the display panel select the Manual or Pressure Cook function.
11. Use the + /- keys and program the Pressure pot for 20 minutes.
12. When the time is up, let the pressure naturally release for 15 minutes, then quickly release the remaining pressure.
13. In a small bowl, mix 1/4 cup of Pressure pot juices and corn-starch.
14. Stir into the pot until thickened.
15. Serve hot topped with shredded cheese.

Nutrition:
Calories 405 | Total Fat 14. 2g | Saturated Fat 9. 8g | Cholesterol 62mg | Sodium 1443mg | Total Carbohydrate 56. 1g | Dietary Fiber 5. 2g |, Total Sugars 8g | Protein 16. 1g

Pasta Puttanesca

Preparation Time: 05 minutes | Cooking Time: 25 minutes | Servings: 2

Ingredients:

- 1 teaspoon garlic powder
- ½ cup pasta sauce
- 2 cups of water
- 2 cups dried rigatoni
- 1/8 teaspoon crushed red pepper flakes
- 1/2 cup pitted Kalamata olives sliced
- ½ teaspoon fine sea salt
- 1/4 teaspoon ground black pepper
- 1 teaspoon grated lemon zest
- ½ cup broccoli

Directions:

1. Combine all of the ingredients in the inner cooking pot and stir to coat the pasta.
2. Lock the lid into place and turn the valve to −Sealing.
3. Select Manual or Pressure Cook and adjust the pressure to High.

4. Set the time for 5 minutes.

5. When cooking ends, carefully turn the valve to —Venting‖ to quickly release the pressure. Unlock and remove the lid.

6. Serve hot.

Nutrition:

Calories 383 | Total Fat 4. 2g | Saturated Fat 0. 9g | Cholesterol 1mg | Sodium 1269mg | Total Carbohydrate 73. 8g | Dietary Fiber 5g | Total Sugars 9g | Protein 12. 4g

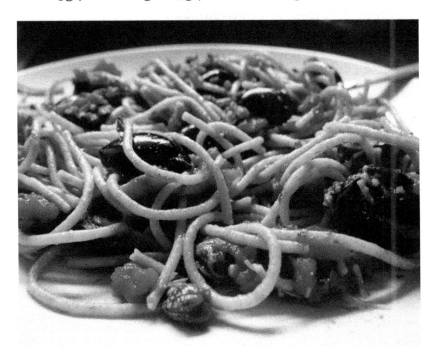

Basil-Coconut Peas and Broccoli

Preparation Time: 05 minutes | Cooking Time: 25 minutes | Servings: 2

Ingredients:

- 1 cup of coconut milk
- 1cup basil
- 1 bell pepper seeded and cut into chunks
- 1 leek green part only, cut into chunks
- 1 teaspoon garlic powder
- ¼ teaspoon salt
- ½ cup of water
- 1 cup noodles
- 1 cup green peas
- ½ cup broccoli florets

Directions:

1. In a blender add the coconut milk, basil, bell pepper, leek, garlic powder, and salt. Blend until smooth.
2. Pour the sauce into the inner pot and add the water.
3. Select Sauté and adjust to High heat.
4. just to a simmer, then turn the Pressure pot off.

5. Break up the noodles into 3 or 4 pieces and place them in the pot in a single layer as much as possible.

6. Layer the broccoli over the noodles.

7. Lock the lid into place.

8. Select Pressure Cook or Manual, and adjust the pressure to Low and the time to 25 minutes.

9. After cooking, quickly release the pressure.

10. Unlock the lid.

11. Gently stir the mixture until the broccoli and peas are coated with sauce.

12. Ladle into bowls and serve immediately.

Nutrition:

Calories 499 | Total Fat 31g | Saturated Fat 25. 8g | Cholesterol 23mg | Sodium 337mg | Total Carbohydrate 49. 2g | Dietary Fiber 10g | Total Sugars 12. 4g | Protein 12. 8g

Spaghetti Squash with Mushroom Sauce Pasta

Preparation Time: 05 minutes | Cooking Time: 25 minutes | Servings: 2

Ingredients:

- ½ tablespoon avocado oil
- 1 cup mushrooms
- 1 cloves garlic minced
- 1/8 cup finely chopped onion
- ¼ cup crushed tomatoes
- 1 teaspoon Italian seasoning blend
- 1 teaspoon garlic powder
- ½ teaspoon dried basil
- ½ teaspoon of sea salt
- ½ teaspoon ground black pepper
- 1/4 cup vegetable broth
- 1 bay leaf
- 1 cup spaghetti squash washed and dried
- 1 tablespoon tomato paste
- 1 tablespoon grated Parmesan cheese
- 1 tablespoon fresh parsley

Directions:

1. Select Sauté (Normal), once the pot is hot, add the avocado oil, mushrooms, garlic, and onions.
2. Sauté, stirring continuously, for about 5 minutes or until the mushrooms are browned.
3. Add the crushed tomatoes, Italian seasoning, garlic powder, basil, sea salt, black pepper, and vegetable broth to the pot.
4. Using a wooden spoon, stir and scrape the bottom of the pot to loosen any browned bits.
5. Add the bay leaf.
6. Using a paring knife, pierce the spaghetti squash 4 or 5 times on each side to create holes for venting the steam.
7. Place the squash in the pot and on top of the sauce.
8. Cover, lock the lid and flip the steam release handle to the sealing position.
9. Select Manual or Pressure Cook (High) and set the cooking time to 8 minutes.
10. When the cooking time is complete, allow the pressure to release naturally for 20 minutes and then quickly release the remaining pressure.
11. Open the lid.
12. Using a slotted spoon, carefully transfer the squash to a cutting board and set aside to cool.
13. Add the tomato paste to the pot and stir.

14. Select Sauté (Less or Low), replace the lid, and let the sauce simmer for 6 minutes.
15. While the sauce is simmering, slice the cooled squash in half and use a spoon to scoop out the seeds.
16. Using a fork, scrape the flesh to create the noodles.
17. Transfer the noodles to a colander to drain, pressing down on the noodles with paper towels to expel any excess moisture.
18. Transfer the noodles to a serving platter.
19. Remove and discard the bay leaf.
20. Ladle the sauce over top of the noodles and garnish with the Parmesan and parsley.
21. Serve warm.

Nutrition:

Calories 115 | Total Fat 4. 1g | Saturated Fat 2. 2g | Cholesterol 10mg | Sodium 893mg | Total Carbohydrate 13. 9 | Dietary Fiber 3. 6g 13% |Total Sugars 6. 1g | Protein 8. 5g

Smoked Tofu and Cherry Tomatoes

Preparation Time: 05 minutes | Cooking Time: 25 minutes | Servings: 2

Ingredients:

- 1 tablespoon coconut oil
- 1 small onion finely diced
- 1/2 cup dry red wine
- 3 cups vegetable broth
- 1 1/4 cups coconut cream
- 1 /2 teaspoon salt
- 1 tablespoon fresh dill
- 1 cup fettuccine pasta, broken in half
- 1 cup cherry or grape tomatoes halved
- 2 cups smoked tofu sliced and cut into bite-sized pieces
- Freshly ground pepper

Directions:

1. Add coconut oil to the Pressure pot.
2. Using the display panel select the Sauté function.
3. Add onion and red wine to the pot and deglaze by using a wooden spoon to scrape any brown

4. bits from the bottom of the pot.
5. Add vegetable broth, coconut cream, salt, and herbs to the pot and stir to combine.
6. Carefully fan the pasta in the pot and ensure it is completely submerged.
7. Add the halved cherry tomatoes in a single layer, do not stir.
8. Turn the pot off by selecting Cancel, then secure the lid, making sure the vent is closed.
9. Using the display panel select the Manual or Pressure Cook function.
10. Use the + /- keys and program the Pressure pot for 5 minutes.
11. When the time is up, let the pressure naturally release for 5 minutes, then quickly release the remaining pressure.
12. Gently stir the pasta, breaking up any clumps.
13. Fold in smoked tofu pieces and serve immediately garnished with freshly ground pepper and additional herbs.

Nutrition:

Calories 501 | Total Fat 31g | Saturated Fat 25. 6g | Cholesterol 31mg | Sodium 1182mg | Total Carbohydrate 40g | Dietary Fiber 3. 7g | Total Sugars 9. 7g | Protein 13g

Cheesy Creamy Farfalle

Preparation Time: 05 minutes | Cooking Time: 25 minutes | Servings: 2

Ingredients:

- 1 cup vegetable broth
- ¼ cup coconut cream
- 1 teaspoon garlic powder
- ½ teaspoon salt
- ¼ teaspoon pepper
- 1 cup dried Farfalle pasta
- 1 cup pasta sauce
- ¼ cup goat cheese shredded
- 1 cup mozzarella cheese shredded
- ½ cups fresh kale finely chopped

Directions:

1. Layer vegetable broth, coconut cream, garlic powder, salt, pepper, and Farfalle pasta in that order in the pot-- do not stir.
2. Ensure all pasta is submerged.
3. Secure the lid, making sure the vent is closed.

4. Using the display panel select the Manual or Pressure Cook function.

5. Use the + /- keys and program the Pressure pot for 6 minutes.

6. When the time is up, let the pressure naturally release for 6 minutes, then quickly release the remaining pressure.

7. Stir in the pasta sauce and kale.

8. Add the cheeses, 1/3 cup at a time, stirring until fully melted and incorporated.

9. Serve hot garnished with finely chopped kale

Nutrition:

Calories 365 | Total Fat 15g | Saturated Fat 9. 4g | Cholesterol 12mg | Sodium 1586mg | Total Carbohydrate 44. 3g | Dietary Fiber 5. 4g | Total Sugars 14. 3g | Protein 13. 8g

Basil Pesto Mushrooms Pasta

Preparation Time: 10 minutes | Cooking Time: 22 minutes | Servings: 2

Ingredients:

- 1 tablespoon coconut oil
- ½ teaspoon garlic powder
- ½ cup mushrooms
- ½ cup cherry tomatoes
- 1 cup pasta
- ½ cup basil pesto
- 1/8 bunch fresh mint
- Salt and pepper to taste
- Enough water

Directions:

1. Set Pressure pot to Sauté.
2. Add coconut oil when it gets hot then add garlic powder.
3. Stir regularly.
4. Add mushrooms and cook until about 4 - 5 minutes, cherry tomatoes, basil pesto, fresh mint, salt, and pepper.
5. Add water and pasta.

6. Lock the lid and make sure the vent is closed.

7. Set Pressure pot to Manual or Pressure Cook on High Pressure for 15 minutes.

8. When cooking time ends, release pressure and wait for steam to completely stop before opening the lid.

Nutrition:

Calories 259 | Total Fat 8. 5g | Saturated Fat 6. 1g | Cholesterol 47mg | Sodium 21mg | Total Carbohydrate 38. 1g | Dietary Fiber 1g | Total Sugars 1. 7g | Protein 8. 5g

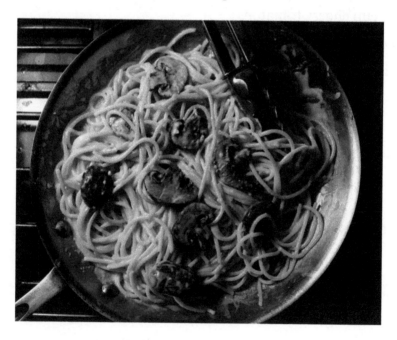

Pressure pot Spaghetti

Preparation Time: 20 minutes | Cooking Time: 15 minutes | Servings: 2

Ingredients:

- 1 tablespoon coconut oil
- ½ cup tofu
- ½ onion, diced
- ½ teaspoon garlic powder
- ¼ teaspoon dried thyme
- ¼ teaspoon dried basil
- ¼ teaspoon salt
- Freshly ground black pepper
- ½ cup jarred spaghetti sauce
- 2 tablespoons tomato paste
- 1 cups vegetable broth
- 2 tablespoon goat cheese, plus extra for serving
- 6 ounces of spaghetti noodles

Directions:

1. Press Sauté on your Pressure pot.
2. Add the coconut oil and tofu to the Pressure pot.
3. Cook for about 3 minutes, stirring and breaking up with a spoon occasionally.

4. Add the chopped onion.

5. Stir, and cook for about 4 minutes.

6. Stir in the garlic powder, thyme, basil, salt, pepper, spaghetti sauce, tomato paste, broth, and goat cheese.

7. Stir very well.

8. Turn off the Pressure pot.

9. Break the noodles in half, and layer them in the tomato mixture, ensuring they are covered by the liquid.

10. Press Pressure Cook and set the timer for 8 minutes.

11. Place the lid on the Pressure pot, and turn the valve to Sealing.

12. When the timer goes off, very carefully do a forced pressure release, cover your hand with a kitchen towel, and gently release the steam.

13. When you hear the float valve drop down, all of the pressure is released.

14. Open the lid to the Pressure pot.

15. It may look like there is a bit too much liquid, but just stir until it all comes together.

16. If it's still too much liquid for you, press Sauté and cook to reduce for 2 minutes.

17. Divide into bowls, and serve topped with more goat cheese.

Nutrition:

Calories 522 | Total Fat 22. 3g | Saturated Fat 13. 9g | Cholesterol 92mg | Sodium 817mg | Total Carbohydrate 54. 9g | Dietary Fiber 2g 7% | Total Sugars 4. 6g | Protein 27g

Mushrooms Creamed Noodles

Preparation Time: 5 minutes | Cooking Time: 20 minutes | Servings: 2

Ingredients:

- ½ cup heavy cream
- 2 cups vegetable broth
- ½ teaspoon dried oregano
- ½ teaspoon garlic minced
- ½ teaspoon red pepper flakes
- 1 cup noodles
- 1 cup mushrooms

Directions:

1. Put ¼ cup of the heavy cream in an Pressure pot.
2. Stir in the broth, oregano, garlic, and red pepper flakes until smooth.
3. Stir in the noodles, then set the block of mushrooms right on top.
4. Lock the lid onto the Pressure pot.
5. Press Pressure Cook on Max Pressure for 3 minutes with the Keep Warm setting off.

6. When the Pressure pot has finished cooking, turn it off and let its pressure return to normal naturally for 1 minute.
7. Then use the Quick-release method to get rid of any residual pressure in the pot.
8. Unlatch the lid and open the cooker.
9. Stir in the remaining 1/4 cup heavy cream.
10. Set the lid askew over the pot and let sit for a couple of minutes so the noodles continue to absorb some of the liquid.
11. Serve hot.

Nutrition:

Calories182 | Total Fat 5. 3g | Saturated Fat 1. 6g | Cholesterol 31mg | Sodium 850mg | Total Carbohydrate 23. 9g | Dietary Fiber 1. 9g | Total Sugars 2g | Protein 10. 2g

Singapore Noodles with Garlic

Preparation Time: 15 minutes | Cooking Time: 20 minutes | Servings: 2

Ingredients:

- 1 cup vermicelli noodles
- ¼ tablespoon hot curry powder
- ½ teaspoon garlic powder
- ½ teaspoon ginger powder
- 1 tablespoon olive oil
- ½ bunch spinach
- 1 medium carrot
- ½ cup green cabbage
- ½ green onions
- 1/8 cup soy sauce
- 1 teaspoon sesame oil
- 1 teaspoon chili garlic sauce, optional

Directions:

1. Place the dry vermicelli noodles in a bowl and cover with room temperature water.
2. Let it soak for 15 minutes.

3. Drain in a colander after they have soaked and are softened.
4. Return the noodles to the bowl, cut the noodles into pieces (approximately 6 inches in length) to facilitate stir-frying later.
5. Sprinkle the noodles with curry powder and toss to coat.
6. Set noodles aside.
7. In the Pressure pot inner pot, place the heated olive oil. add the garlic powder and ginger powder.
8. Stir fry very briefly (1 minute or less) then add all of the vegetables.
9. Stir fry the vegetables until they just begin to soften.
10. Add sesame oil, water noodles, soy sauce, salt, pepper, and chili garlic sauce.
11. Lock the lid and make sure the vent is closed.
12. Set Pressure pot to Manual or Pressure Cook on High Pressure for 15 minutes.
13. When cooking time ends, release pressure and wait for steam to completely stop before opening the lid.
14. Serve.

Nutrition:

Calories 244 | Total Fat 11. 5g | Saturated Fat 1. 7g | Cholesterol 23mg | Sodium 1036mg | Total Carbohydrate 30. 2g | Dietary Fiber 4. 8g | Total Sugars 3. 3g | Protein 7. 9g

Garlic Noodles

Preparation Time: 10 minutes | Cooking Time: 15 minutes | Servings: 2

Ingredients:

- ½ cup spaghetti
- 1 cup of coconut milk
- 1 tablespoon goat cheese
- 2 tablespoon butter
- 1 teaspoon soy sauce
- 1 tablespoon honey
- 1 tablespoon oyster sauce
- 1 teaspoon olive oil
- Enough water
- Salt to taste

Directions:

1. Add the oyster sauce, honey, soy sauce, and olive oil to a bowl and stir until combined.
2. Add spaghetti, water, and salt to Pressure pot.
3. Place the lid on the pot and lock it into place to seal.
4. Pressure Cook on High Pressure for 4 minutes.

5. Use Quick Pressure Release.

6. Stir milk into Spaghetti and then stir in the cheeses until melted and combined.

7. Add sauce mix well.

Nutrition:

Calories 239 | Total Fat 11. 2g | Saturated Fat 6. 1g | Cholesterol 58mg | Sodium 199mg | Total Carbohydrate 29. 5g | Dietary Fiber 0. 1g | Total Sugars 3. 6g | Protein 5. 6g

Green Goddess Pasta

Preparation Time: 10 minutes | Cooking Time: 15 minutes | Servings: 2

Ingredients:

- 1 tablespoon butter
- 1 cup mushrooms, sliced
- ½ tablespoon garlic powder
- 1 cup pasta vegetable
- 2 cups vegetable broth
- ½ cup baby kale
- ½ cup peas
- ½ cup coconut cream, cubed
- ¼ cup pesto sauce
- ¼ cup grated goat cheese

Directions:

1. Add butter to the Pressure pot, hit —Sauté‖ and once the butter is melted and sizzled, add in the mushrooms and cook for 2-3 minutes until they begin lightly brown.
2. Then, add the garlic powder and stir for another 2 minutes.

3. Next, add in the pasta vegetable and broth.

4. Top off with the kale and secure the lid and hit —Keep Warm/Cancel‖ and then hit —Manual‖ or —Pressure Cook‖ High Pressure for 6 minutes.

5. Quick-release when done.

6. Stir in the peas.

7. Then, add in the coconut cream and pesto, and goat cheese and stir for about 2 minutes more until the cheese is completely melted into the sauce.

8. to a serving dish and top with grated goat cheese.

9. Enjoy!

Nutrition:

Calories 677 | Total Fat 43. 4g | Saturated Fat 20. 4g | Cholesterol 137mg | Sodium 1203mg | Total Carbohydrate 48. 6g | Dietary Fiber 3. 2g | Total Sugars 6. 1g | Protein 24. 4g

Simply Kale Lasagna

Preparation Time: 15 minutes | Cooking Time: 45 minutes | Servings: 2

Ingredients:

- 1 cup pasta sauce
- 1/8 cup water
- 1 large egg
- 2-1/2 cups shredded Italian cheese blend divided
- 1 cup ricotta cheese
- ½ cup kale
- 1 cup oven-ready (no-boil) lasagna noodles

Directions:

1. Add 1/2 cup sauce into a pan.
2. Transfer the remaining sauce to a bowl and stir in water.
3. In a large bowl, whisk the egg.
4. Stir in 1-3/4 cups Italian cheese and ricotta blend them.
5. Layer one-quarter of the noodles on top of the sauce in the pan, breaking noodles as needed to evenly cover the sauce.

6. Top with one-third of the cheese mixture with kale, then one quarter of the sauce.

7. Continue with two more layers each of noodles, cheese mixture, and sauce, gently pressing down on the noodles between each layer.

8. Finish with a layer of noodles and a layer of sauce.

9. Add 1 1/2 cups water and the steam rack to the Pressure pot. Place the baking pan on the rack.

10. Close and lock the lid and turn the steam release handle to Sealing.

11. Set your Pressure pot to Pressure Cook on High for 14 minutes.

12. When the cooking time is done, press Cancel and turn the steam release handle to Venting.

13. When the float valve drops down, remove the lid.

14. Sprinkle with the remaining Italian cheese blend.

15. Close and lock the lid and let it stand for 10 minutes or until the cheese is melted.

16. Using the handles of the rack, carefully remove the rack and pan.

17. Let Lasagna stand for 10 minutes.

18. Cut into wedges.

Nutrition:

Calories 491 | Total Fat 22. 4g | Saturated Fat 11. 3g | Cholesterol 156mg | Sodium 898mg | Total Carbohydrate 43. 8g | Dietary Fiber 4. 3g | Total Sugars 12. 1g | Protein 29. 5g

Mozzarella Lemon Pasta

Preparation Time: 05 minutes | Cooking Time: 45 minutes | Servings: 2

Ingredients:

- ½ tablespoon olive oil
- ½ teaspoon garlic powder
- 2 cups vegetable broth
- Zest of one lemon
- 1 tablespoon lemon juice divided
- 1 cup ziti noodles
- ½ cup grated/shredded mozzarella cheese
- ½ cup coconut cream
- Salt and pepper to taste
- ½ tablespoon cornstarch
- 1 tablespoon cold water
- 1 tablespoon finely chopped parsley for serving
- Additional mozzarella for serving

Directions:

1. Add olive oil to the Pressure pot.
2. Using the display panel select the Sauté function.

3. Add garlic powder, vegetable broth, lemon zest, and lemon juice to the pot and deglaze by using a wooden spoon to scrape any brown bits from the bottom of the pot.

4. Break noodles in half and fan across the bottom of the pot, making sure all noodles are submerged.

5. Turn the pot off by selecting Cancel, then secure the lid, making sure the vent is closed.

6. Using the display panel select the Manual or Pressure Cook function.

7. Use the + /- keys and program the Pressure pot for 3 minutes.

8. When the time is up, let the pressure naturally release for 10 minutes, then quickly release the remaining pressure.

9. Stir, breaking up any pasta clumps, and allow to cool slightly.

10. Add mozzarella cheese, coconut cream, and remaining lemon juice.

11. Add salt and pepper to taste.

12. In a small bowl, mix cornstarch and cold water. Stir into the pot until thickened, returning to Sauté mode as needed.

13. Serve warm topped finely chopped parsley and additional mozzarella.

Nutrition:

Calories 331 | Total Fat 21g | Saturated Fat 14. 4g | Cholesterol 4mg | Sodium 895mg | Total Carbohydrate 26. 3g | Dietary Fiber 2. 5g | Total Sugars 4g | Protein 12g

Grilled Tempeh with Green Beans

Preparation Time: 15-30 minutes | Cooking Time: 15 minutes | Servings: 4

Ingredients:

- 1 tbsp plant butter, melted
- 1 lb tempeh, sliced into 4 pieces
- 1 lb green beans, trimmed
- Salt and black pepper to taste
- 2 sprigs thyme
- 2 tbsp olive oil
- 1 tbsp pure corn syrup
- 1 lemon, juiced

Directions:

1. Preheat a grill pan over medium heat and brush with the plant butter.
2. Season the tempeh and green beans with salt, black pepper, and place the thyme in the pan.

3. Grill the tempeh and green beans on both sides until golden brown and tender, 10 minutes.
4. Transfer to serving plates.
5. In a small bowl, whisk the olive oil, corn syrup, lemon juice, and drizzle all over the food.
6. Serve warm.

Nutrition:

• Calories 352 | Fats 22. 5g | Carbs 21. 8g | Protein 22. 6g

Creamy Fettuccine with Peas

Preparation Time: 15-30 minutes | Cooking Time: 25 minutes | Servings: 4

Ingredients:

- 16 oz whole-wheat fettuccine
- Salt and black pepper to taste
- ¾ cup flax milk
- ½ cup cashew butter, room temperature
- 1 tbsp olive oil
- 2 garlic cloves, minced
- 1 ½ cups frozen peas
- ½ cup chopped fresh basil

Directions:

1. Add the fettuccine and 10 cups of water to a large pot, and cook over medium heat until al dente, 10 minutes.
2. Drain the pasta through a colander and set aside. In a bowl, whisk the flax milk, cashew butter, and salt until smooth. Set aside.
3. Heat the olive oil in a large skillet and sauté the garlic until fragrant, 30 seconds. Mix in the peas, fettuccine,

and basil. Toss well until the pasta is well-coated in the sauce and season with some black pepper.

4. Dish the food and serve warm.

Nutrition:

• Calories 654 | Fats 23. 7g | Carbs 101. 9g | Protein 18. 2g

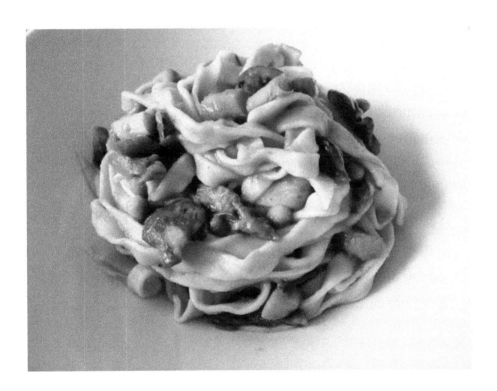

Buckwheat Cabbage Rolls

Preparation Time: 15-30 minutes | Cooking Time: 30 minutes | Servings: 4

Ingredients:

- 2 tbsp plant butter
- 2 cups extra-firm tofu, pressed and crumbled
- ½ medium sweet onion, finely chopped
- 2 garlic cloves, minced
- Salt and black pepper to taste
- 1 cup buckwheat groats
- 1 ¾ cups vegetable stock
- 1 bay leaf
- 2 tbsp chopped fresh cilantro + more for garnishing
- 1 head Savoy cabbage, leaves separated (scraps kept)
- 1 (23 oz) canned chopped tomatoes

Directions:

1. Melt the plant butter in a large bowl and cook the tofu until golden brown, 8 minutes. Stir in the onion and garlic until softened and fragrant, 3 minutes. Season with

salt, black pepper, and mix in the buckwheat, bay leaf, and vegetable stock.

2. Close the lid, allow boiling, and then simmer until all the liquid is absorbed. Open the lid; remove the bay leaf, adjust the taste with salt, black pepper, and mix in the cilantro.

3. Lay the cabbage leaves on a flat surface and add 3 to 4 tablespoons of the cooked buckwheat onto each leaf. Roll the leaves to firmly secure the filling.

4. Pour the tomatoes with juices into a medium pot, season with a little salt, black pepper, and lay the cabbage rolls in the sauce. Cook over medium heat until the cabbage softens, 5 to 8 minutes. Turn the heat off and dish the food onto serving plates. Garnish with more cilantro and serve warm.

Nutrition:

Calories 1147 | Fats 112. 9g | Carbs 25. 6g | Protein 23. 8g

Bbq Black Bean Burgers

Preparation Time: 15-30 minutes | Cooking Time: 20 minutes | Servings: 4

Ingredients:

- 3 (15 oz) cans black beans, drained and rinsed
- 2 tbsp whole-wheat flour
- 2 tbsp quick-cooking oats
- ¼ cup chopped fresh basil
- 2 tbsp pure barbecue sauce
- 1 garlic clove, minced
- Salt and black pepper to taste
- 4 whole-grain hamburger buns, split
- For topping:
- Red onion slices
- Tomato slices
- Fresh basil leaves
- Additional barbecue sauce

Directions:

1. In a medium bowl, mash the black beans and mix in the flour, oats, basil, barbecue sauce, garlic salt, and black

pepper until well combined. Mold 4 patties out of the mixture and set aside.

2. Heat a grill pan to medium heat and lightly grease with cooking spray.

3. Cook the bean patties on both sides until light brown and cooked through, 10 minutes.

4. Place the patties between the burger buns and top with the onions, tomatoes, basil, and some barbecue sauce.

5. Serve warm.

Nutrition:

Calories 589 | Fats 17. 7g | Carbs 80. 9g | Protein 27. 9g

Paprika & Tomato Pasta Primavera

Preparation Time: 15-30 minutes | Cooking Time: 25 minutes | Servings: 4

Ingredients:

- 2 tbsp olive oil
- 8 oz whole-wheat fedelini
- ½ tsp paprika
- 1 small red onion, sliced
- 2 garlic cloves, minced
- 1 cup dry white wine
- Salt and black pepper to taste
- 2 cups cherry tomatoes, halved
- 3 tbsp plant butter, cut into ½-in cubes
- 1 lemon, zested and juiced
- 1 cup packed fresh basil leaves

Directions:

1. Heat the olive oil in a large pot and mix in the fedelini, paprika, onion, garlic, and stir-fry for

2. 2-3 minutes.
3. Mix in the white wine, salt, and black pepper. Cover with water. Cook until the water absorbs
4. and the fedelini al dente, 5 minutes. Mix in the cherry tomatoes, plant butter, lemon zest,
5. lemon juice, and basil leaves.
6. Dish the food and serve warm.

Nutrition:

Calories 380 kcal |Fats 24. 1g | Carbs 33. 7g | Protein 11. 2g

Green Lentil Stew with Brown Rice

Preparation Time: 15-30 minutes | Cooking Time: 50 minutes | Servings: 4

Ingredients:

For the stew:

- 2 tbsp olive oil
- 1 lb tempeh, cut into cubes
- Salt and black pepper to taste
- 1 tsp chili powder
- 1 tsp onion powder
- 1 tsp cumin powder
- 1 tsp garlic powder
- 1 yellow onion, chopped
- 2 celery stalks, chopped
- 2 carrots diced
- 4 garlic cloves, minced
- 2 cups vegetable broth
- 1 tsp oregano
- 1 cup green lentils, rinsed
- ¼ cup chopped tomatoes
- 1 lime, juiced

For the brown rice:

- 1 cup of brown rice
- 1 cup of water
- Salt to taste

Directions:

- Heat the olive oil in a large pot, season the tempeh with salt, black pepper, and cook in the oil until brown, 10 minutes.
- Stir in the chili powder, onion powder, cumin powder, garlic powder, and cook until fragrant, 1 minute. Mix in the onion, celery, carrots, garlic, and cook until softened. Pour in the vegetable broth, oregano, green lentils, tomatoes, and green chilies.
- Cover the pot and cook until the tomatoes soften and the stew reduces by half, 10 to 15 minutes. Open the lid, adjust the taste with salt, black pepper, and mix in the lime juice. Dish the stew and serve warm with the brown rice.
- Meanwhile, as the stew cooks, add the brown rice, water, and salt to a medium pot. Cook over medium heat until the rice is tender and the water is absorbed for about 15 to 25 minutes.

Nutrition:

Calories 1305 kcal | Fats 130. 9g | Carbs 25. 1g | Protein 24. 3g

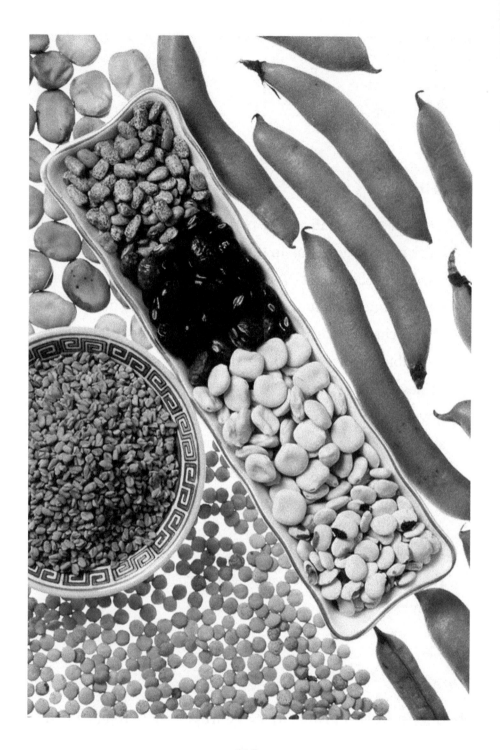

Lightning Source UK Ltd.
Milton Keynes UK
UKHW020644010621
384724UK00004B/40